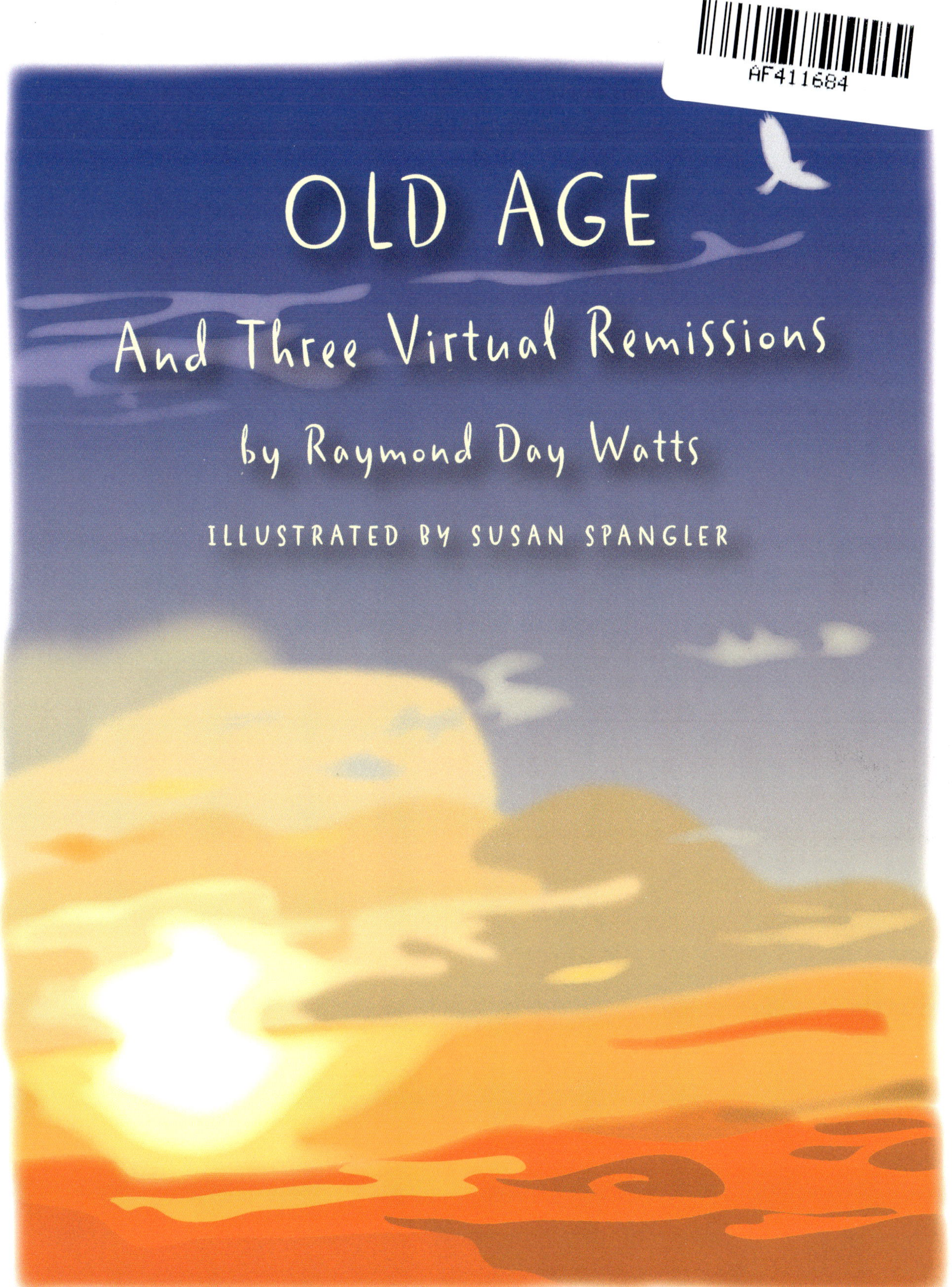

EXPLICIT ADULT CONTENT

Not Suitable for Children

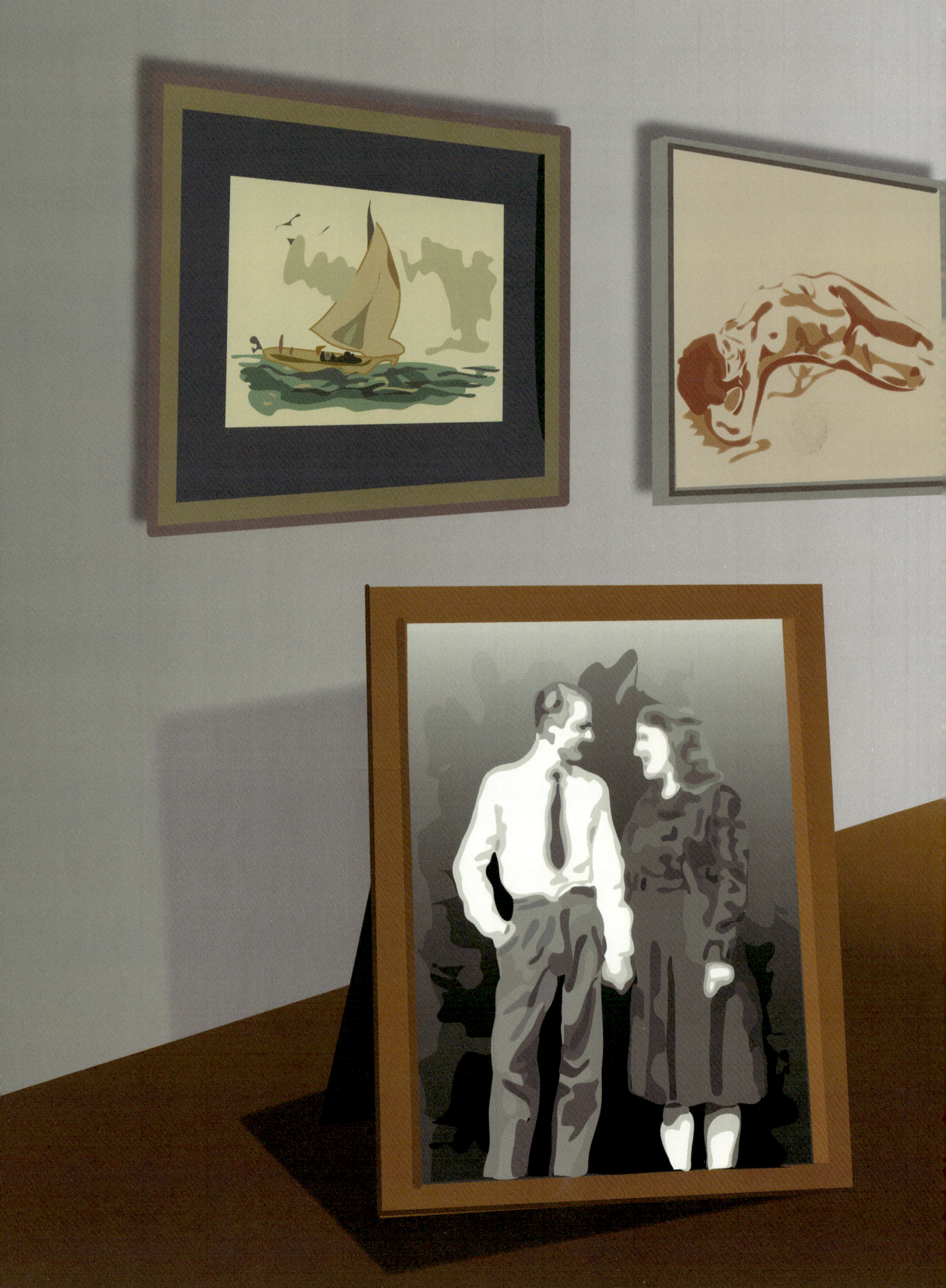

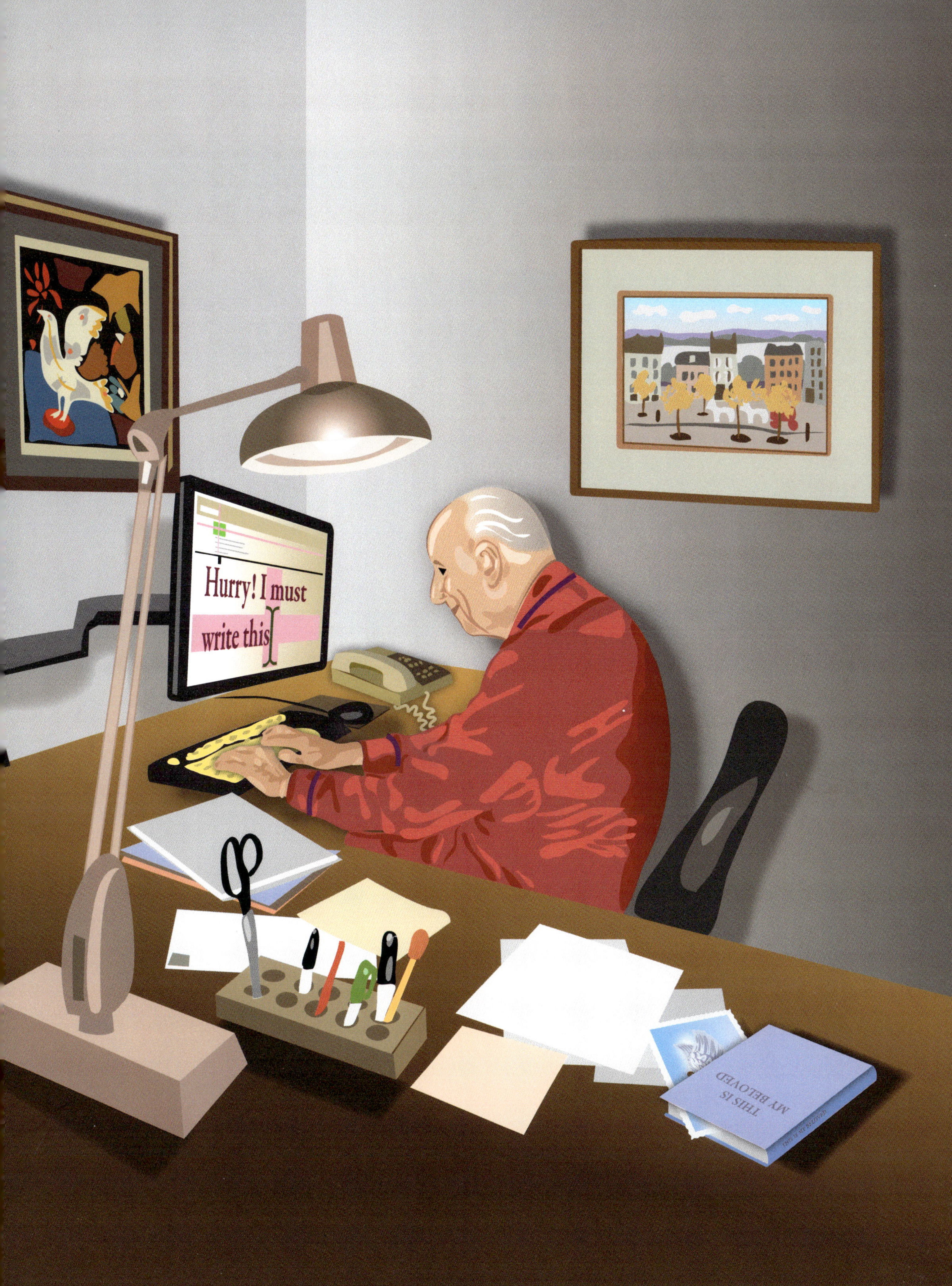

Hurry! I must write this
THIS IS
MY BELOVED

Old Age and Three Virtual Remissions
by Raymond Day Watts
www.oldage3.com

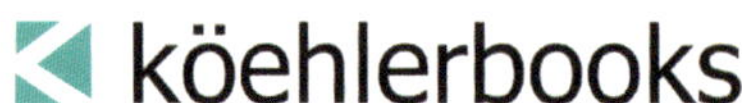

Published by Koehler Books
210 60th Street, Virginia Beach, Virginia 23451
www.koehlerbooks.com

Printed in the United States

____

ISBN 978-0-9835013-5-0

For more information about this book and all other inquiries,
contact John Koehler, 757-289-6006, john@koehlerbooks.com

Illustration and Book Design by Susan Spangler

PUBLISHER'S NOTE

This is a book about hope and truth. It is not often that we hear such passion and clarity from an octogenarian, as our society tends to put seniors far, far away in places where they are out of mind and out of sight. But the truth is that their lives are as vital and amazing and filled with love and desire as they were during the days of their youth. Ray Watts has expressed his life in this book with complete honesty as he tells us the story of his wife, medical ailments and how his dreams ultimately fulfilled his emotional and physical needs. Some of the illustrations are also quite honest and revealing, but they were deemed necessary in order to fulfill the story of the author. They are beautifully rendered with exquisite detail by the illustrator and friend of the author, Susan Spangler. This is a book for grown ups with open minds, and is not intended for children. We sincerely hope that you will enjoy this book and accept it in the same manner it was given by the author and illustrator: with love, truth and integrity.

For a multitude of memories happy and sad

I dedicate this little book to my wife

Anne Pennybacker (Penny) Watts

September 6, 1927 – June 28, 2009

Wedding June 18, 1948

with love

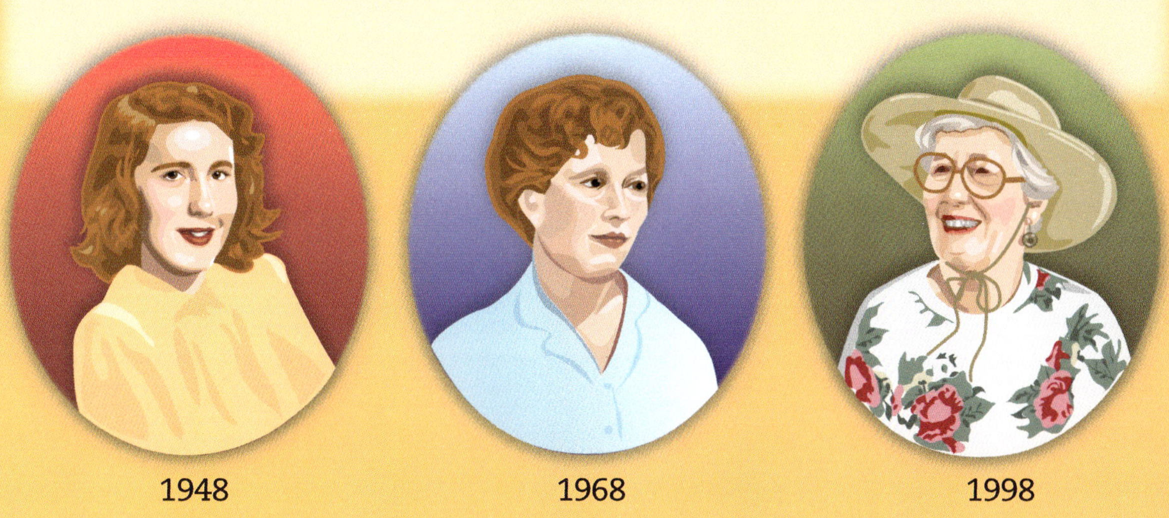

1948   1968   1998

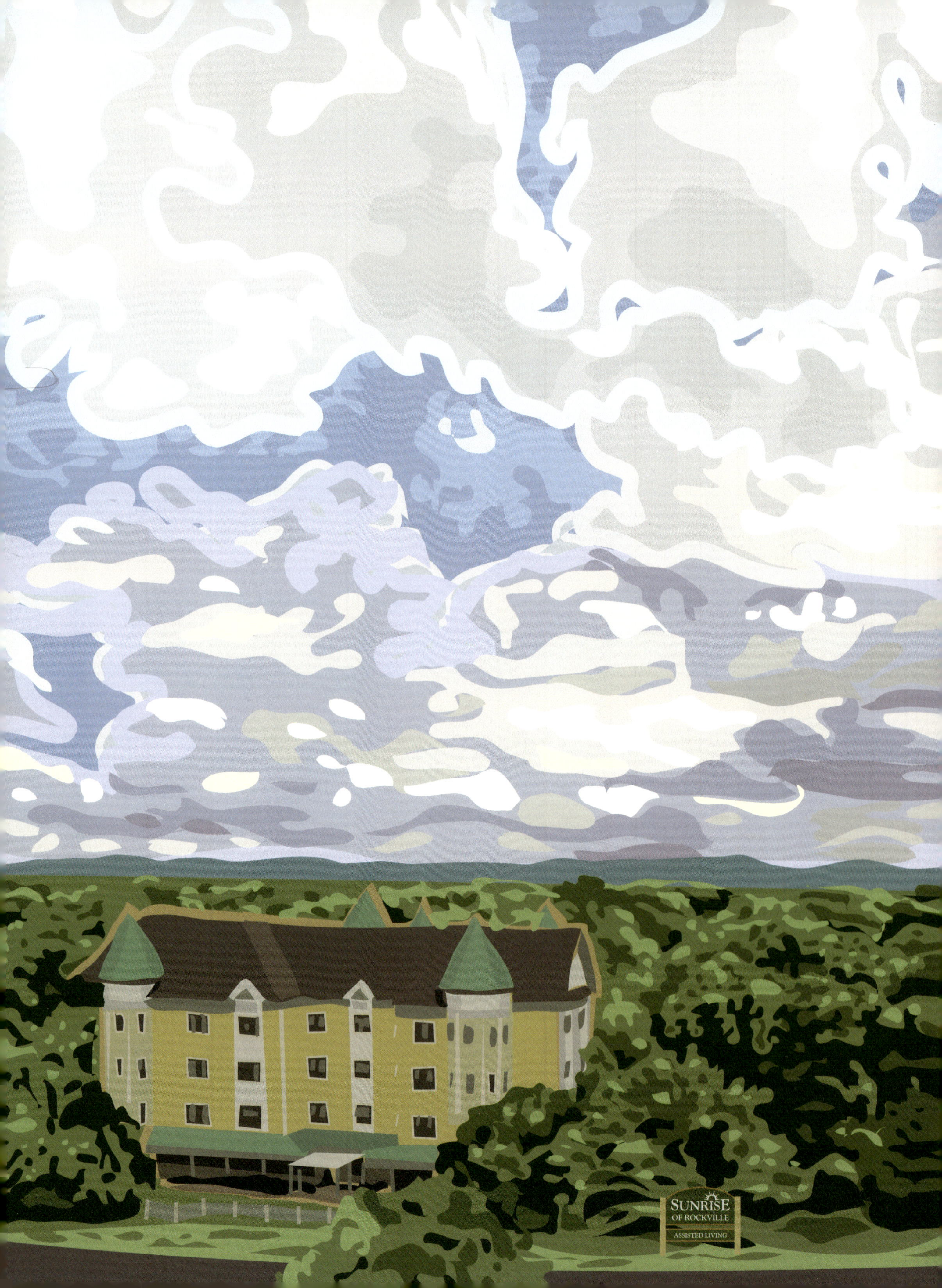

SUNRISE
OF ROCKVILLE
ASSISTED LIVING

It's All True! (mostly)

In November 2001 a very good neurologist diagnosed my wife Penny's increasing forgetfulness as "probable" Alzheimer's disease. I'm told that no diagnostician will leave out the "probable" until the patient has died and had an autopsy; but the symptoms are soon enough plenty clear to the family.

In the fall of 2002 my urologist told me, after a biopsy, that a small new lump in my prostate was cancerous. I was given a choice: watchful waiting, or an operation to implant radioactive seeds in the prostate to kill the cancer. To my undying regret, I chose the second alternative. In January 2003 I was given a drug, Lupron, to shrink the prostate before the operation.

I was warned that it would render me impotent "for about six months." I gulped but said OK. The drug was injected, the prostate shrank, the operation—a duet surgery which the urologist performed in tandem with a radiotherapy oncologist—took place in May. As advertised, the wee cancer was annihilated; but, soon after the surgery on the advice of both surgeons, I took a Lupron booster shot. In January 2004, not as advertised, the Lupron impotence was still in full sway—and, in 2011, it still is.

In March 2004 Penny's condition had advanced to a point where I, even with a great care-giving helper named Sandra Desonier, could no longer handle her at home. She moved, on my insistence and over her objection, into a Sunrise assisted living facility.

The oxymoronic name of that chain, "Sunrise," is compounded by the cute designation of their dementia ward: the "Reminiscence Neighborhood." By the winter of 2006–07 her disease was so far along that she had stopped resenting the place and had become the Ms. Sunshine of the floor, loved by all the staff and many of the other residents for her bright smile and cheery manner. She had in fact become a satisfied resident and I a satisfied customer of Sunrise of Rockville.

In February 2007 I was feeling good enough, on balance, to begin a poem titled "A well-heeled man, 82, considers OLD AGE," with the lines, "Well sure, it beats the alternative—so far" and end it with "I am—happy."

A recitation of that poem by me at the second semi-annual Poetry Coffee House of the Unitarian Universalist Church of Rockville, Maryland, was so well received that I was called upon to repeat the performance at a Sunday worship service.

Alzheimer's is a terminal disease, and Penny reached the terminal in June 2009. Her illness before and Lupron after January 2003 had obliterated my sex life; but, in January of 2010, I had a dream that amounted to a virtual semi-remission from impotence.

Excited, I wrote another poem about that, which I recited, following a reprise of the Old Age poem, at the fifth semi-annual UUCR Poetry Coffee House in April of that year. The new poem, I felt, needed a caveat, and I gave one:

"To me, the most powerful and sad line of the Old Age poem is: 'but I'll never again know erection and orgasm.'

Well, early one morning last January I made an amazing discovery. When I'm asleep and dreaming and have eaten a lot of vitamin C, that line can become only half true. I had a dream that starred a full, long-lasting erection, being used for the most favored purpose of erections. When I woke up I was so excited I had to write a poem about it immediately.

It contains no dirty words but does frankly mention human private parts, their names, functions and fits. Some will see such a poem as a dirty old man's pornography or at best terrible taste; but I disagree. I see it as a deprived old man's clean exultation over a brief, virtual semi-remission from impotence. But if you think my poem might embarrass or offend you, or you have young kids with you, I won't be embarrassed or offended if you want to duck out to the lobby until it's over. ALL ESCAPE THAT WANT TO ESCAPE! No takers? OK, you were warned. Here goes."

Exactly one week after that performance I had another dream starring another virtual remission, this one from both halves of my impotence. While it was still fresh I again captured that memory in another poem. This book gratifies my urge to publish all three poems together, with pictures. But months later, in January 2011, with work on the book well along, I had another dream good enough to call forth another poem. It seemed to put an exclamation point on all that had preceded it.

I open my little book with a Prologue: a letter I wrote to Mom and Dad on February 24, 1948, announcing with jubilation Penny's acceptance of my marriage proposal. The best sex, holy sex, be it real or virtual, is between two people who share true love. This letter is my evidence that we did.

Oh yes, just a note more, about the pictures on pages 14 and 19. When my boyhood chum Rob (Robin) Kidd and I reported for our military physicals in 1943, I was 1A and drafted; he was 4F and was not drafted. We each had some reciprocal envy. On the Army's motion, I learned how to be an Infantry rifleman. On his own motion, Robin went on to the U.S. Merchant Marine Academy at King's Point and learned how to be a skipper on a merchant ship.

In one of our infrequent meetings during or just after World War II, Merchant Captain Kidd showed Infantry Private First Class Watts some wondrous souvenirs from Naples: iterations in various forms, from picture postcard to silver watch fob, of the classic winged phallus, a revered fertility charm and sex symbol of ancient Pompeii and other Mediterranean cultures. A colored postcard of the beloved flying penis in a blue sky with two naked young lovers riding it made an impression on me, the youth that I, the old man, cannot forget. The memory of that card fuses with the happiest memories of life and sex with my wife.

But we live in twenty-first century America, not first century Pompeii, and in deference to contemporary tastes and taboos, our conveyance through rapturous skies on page 19 has been changed from a winged phallus to a dove. If you are as nostalgic for Pompeiian tastes as I am, you can use your imagination to change it back.

—R.D.W.

June 1, 2011

3

Prologue

At age 23, on February 24, 1948, I used the old Corona portable
typewriter that was my companion all through college and
the war to type a joyful letter, sent Special Delivery, to
Mr. and Mrs. T. R. Watts, Forest Hills, Pennsylvania.
What follows is its mercifully abridged text.

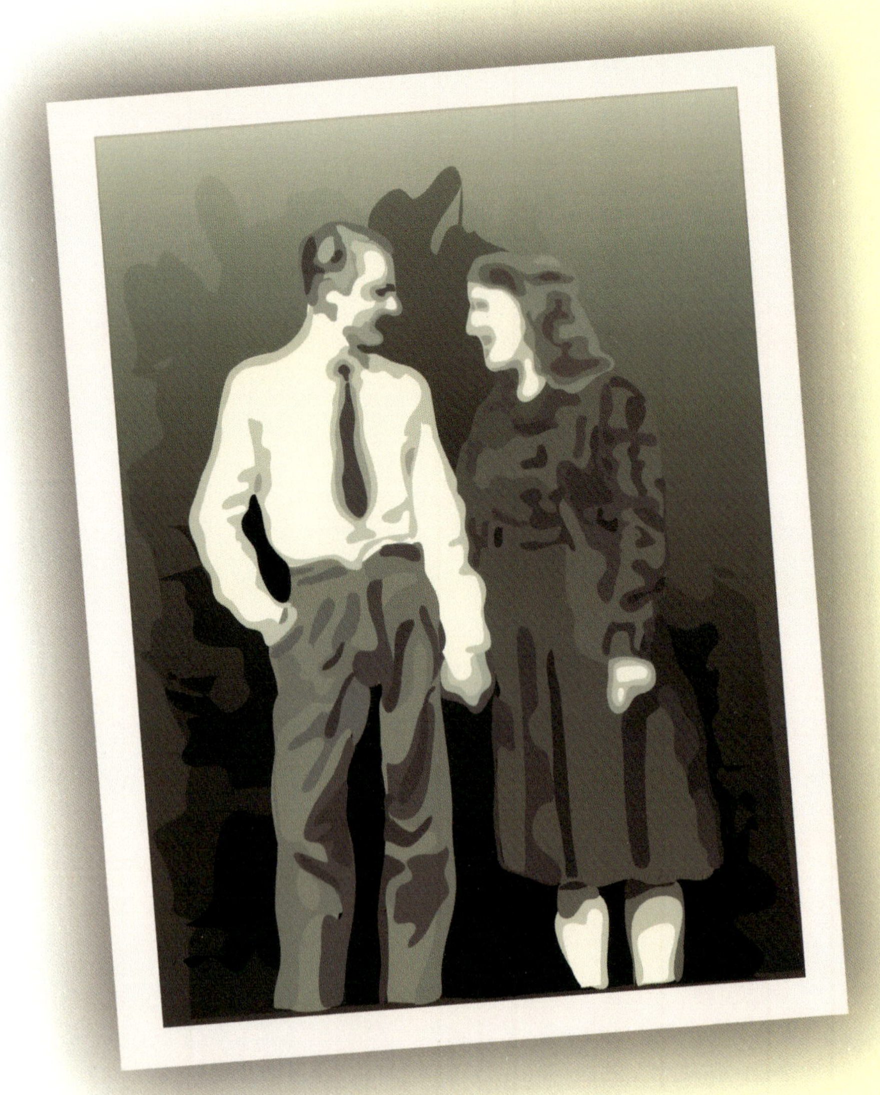

The Pen House at Mills

Tuesday, Feb. 24, '48

Dearest Mom and Dad,

It's happened. The Wonderful, Amazing, Awesomely Beautiful Thing has happened. Penny is in love with me, really and truly in love. Excuse me if I sound a little delirious, and don't make too much sense: my eyes seem to have a tendency to mist over now and then, for I am bewildered, nearly dazed with the sheer weight of happiness.

It doesn't usually happen this way, you see, and it's still a little hard to believe and quite overwhelming. How often does it happen …what are the odds…that a guy falls in love and nurses a dream along for eight bleak months, then has the dream come true and the reality proves to be more lovely than the vision?

I don't know exactly what did it, when the subtle sorceries I've so long been weaving in vain suddenly began to click; but gradually, during the last few weeks, my suit has risen perceptibly, almost daily, in her esteem. Over three weeks ago she said she thought she might love me, but wouldn't say she did until she felt quite sure. We went to the concert in Dayton on the 12th, and that night she said she would tell me when she loved me if she thought she'd feel the same way "at 10 o'clock in the morning three weeks from now." Last Friday night, though, and on several incredibly happy occasions since then, she's said it and meant it (one of the things I've always loved about Penny is that she doesn't say things she *doesn't* mean), and with no qualifications. And my patient, plodding

5

feet—which I've been holding to the ground with increasing difficulty of late—have snapped free of the mud with a resounding "Thu-luck!" and I'm now pink clouds from head to toe and as far as the arm can reach, the eye can see and the mind can think.

As of today we are thinking—cautiously, carefully, experimentally; above all, in the daytime!—about getting married when school lets out, or shortly before. It'll take a lot of thinking, and we don't feel that we can make up our minds about it until after spring vacation. The main problem to be mulled over still is: Does Penny really love me in a lifetime, breakfast-together-in-1980 sort of way? As I've told you earlier, she couldn't tell for at least six months; but, three of them are past and spent miles away from me. At this point, however, three or six months sound like seventeen centuries to both of us. Since we're committed to spend the summer working together, we are maddened at the contemplation of spending it as bachelor and maiden.

She *has* known me, and known me very well, for well over a year; it's just this sudden, bewildering "passion" side of our acquaintance which is still new to her, and she has to look it over for awhile and see how it wears, how it looks on her, so to speak, for a few weeks. Soooo, what we think we'll do is just keep these developments under our hats for the rest of this div, and wait until Penny has gone home for that week of spring vacation, talked it over with her folks, and considered things away from me, then make up our minds, or rather hers. I, after all, have long since resolved any doubts of my own: I'll wait for her until 1954 and not a day longer. If, after she gets back, she still feels the way she does now, and has been able to convince her family of her considered sincerity (she anticipates some kick-back there), then we shall certainly examine every possibility of getting married in June.

But enough! I also have utterly formidable heaps of work facing me. Much good 'twill do me, with all my long-range planning, to flunk out of Antioch for having given up all my study time to alternate sessions with Penny on Rohmann's and Lithgow's davenports with lyricising to you about it. To work! Penny and I have decided not to see each other after eight o'clock at night until Saturday. We're too darn likely to forget to do any studying.

I repeat, however, that Penny and I are keeping all these things and pondering them in our hearts until after spring vacation (when I shall doubtless be home for a couple of days, at least, to talk these matters over further with you), so kindly don't spread the word about the family yet. But then, unless I am very much mistaken, you can raise the clarion call as loudly as you like and summon the kinfolk to the nuptials, for I feel as surely optimistic now as I was pessimistic at Christmas; the sun is shining, and all things are fair.

Penny Watts! It sounds kindo' strange to me, silly even…but Penny says she likes it. I'm crazy about it myself.

Love,
Ray

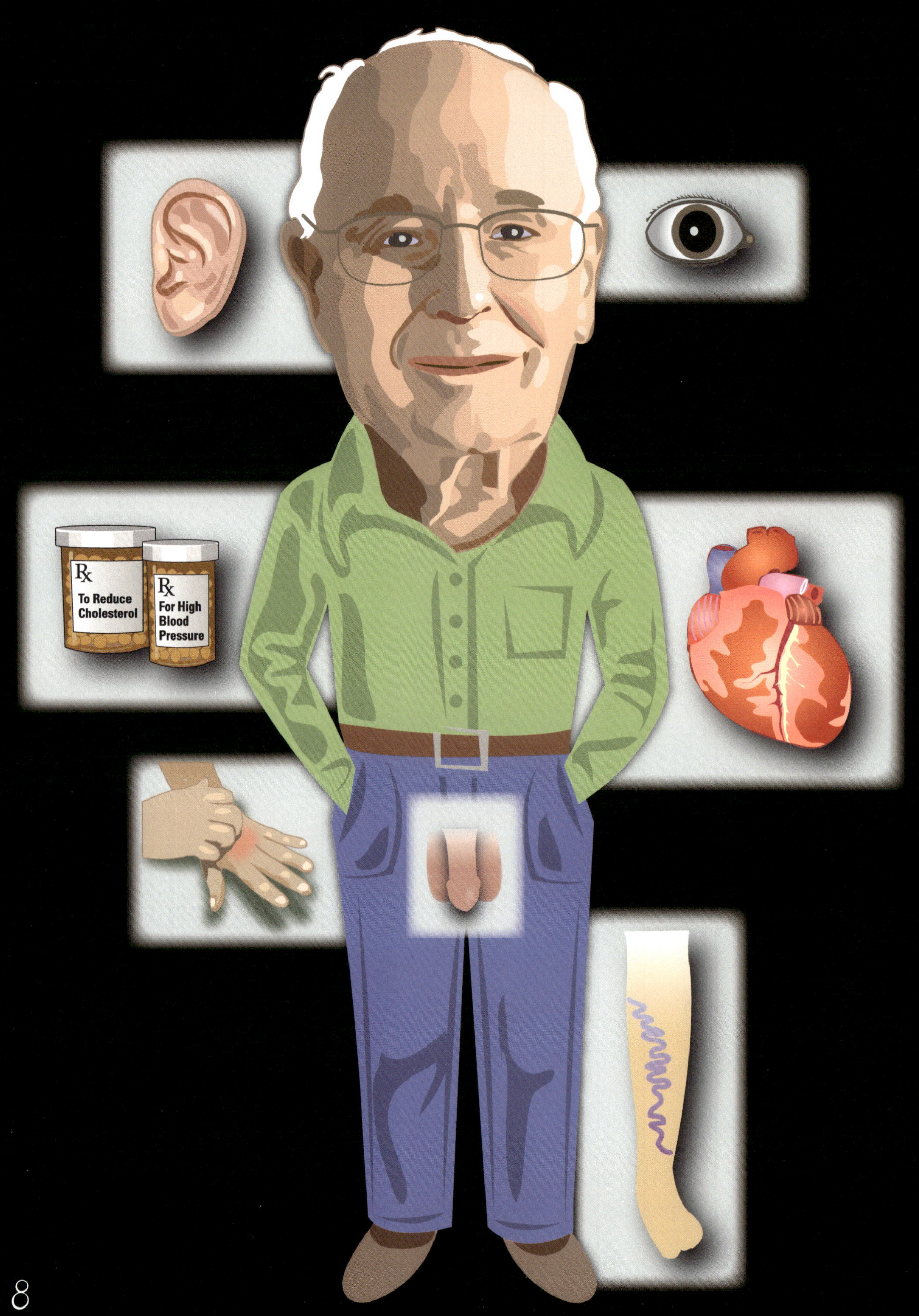
Rx
To Reduce
Cholesterol
Rx
For High
Blood
Pressure

A Well-Heeled Man, 82, Considers
OLD AGE

Well sure, it beats the alternative—

    so far.

But God! What a drag!

The internist, podiatrist, dermatologist, cardiologist—

    bless 'em all—

just within the past ten days

have dealt with

wax in my ears, my varicose veins, assorted itches,

blood pressure and cholesterol.

I'm moving up my date with the ophthalmologist

because my dim vision is getting even dimmer.

The quadruple bypass surgery a few years ago

was a great success.

The prostate surgery the same year

stopped the cancer—

    but I'll never again know erection and orgasm

        and will forevermore wear a diaper twenty-four/seven.

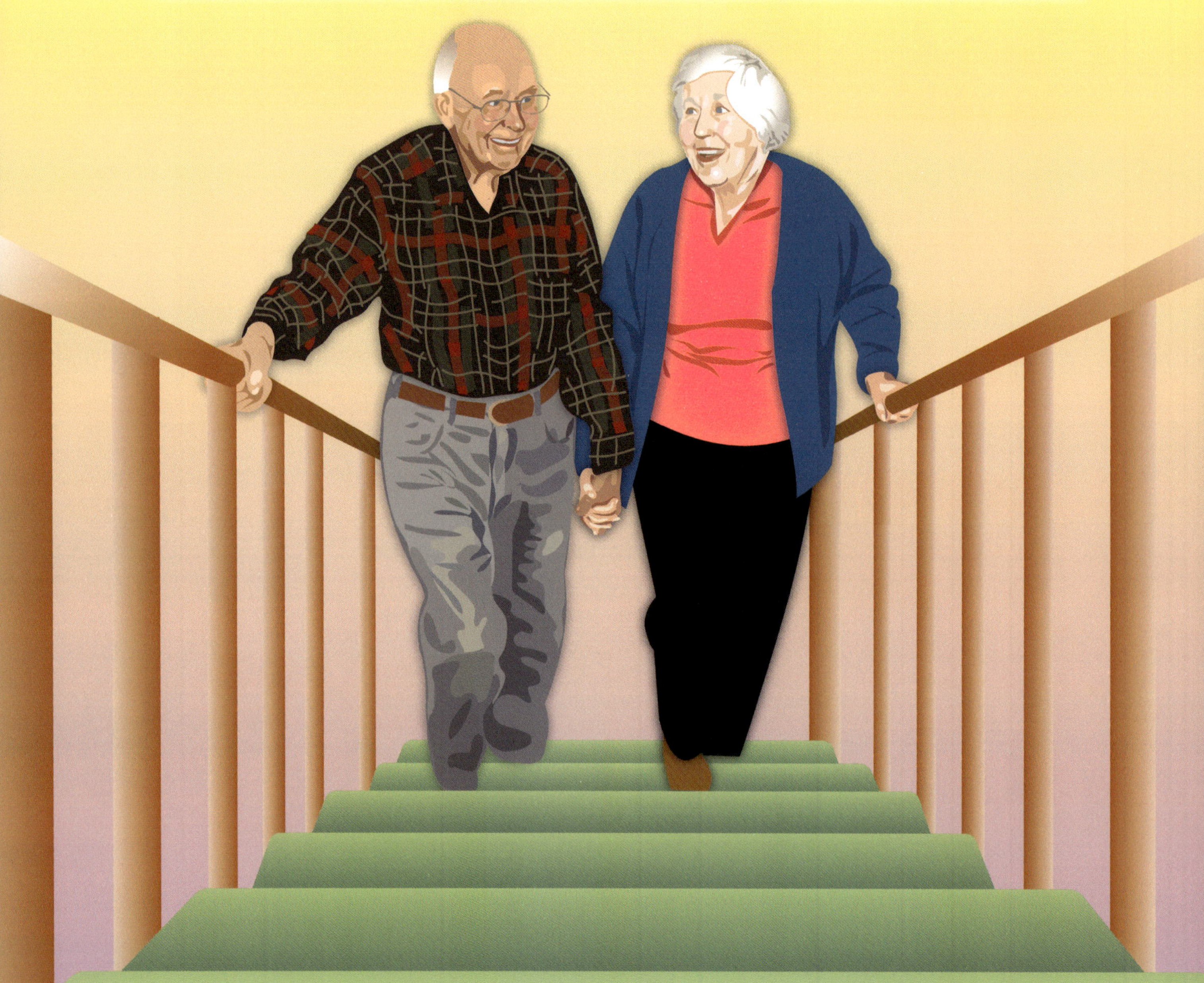

My dear wife of fifty-eight years has Alzheimer's

but greets me joyfully when I visit

the dementia ward

and counts aloud with me the steps between floors,

one to twenty, as we walk them together,

down and up, before sharing the fruit I bring,

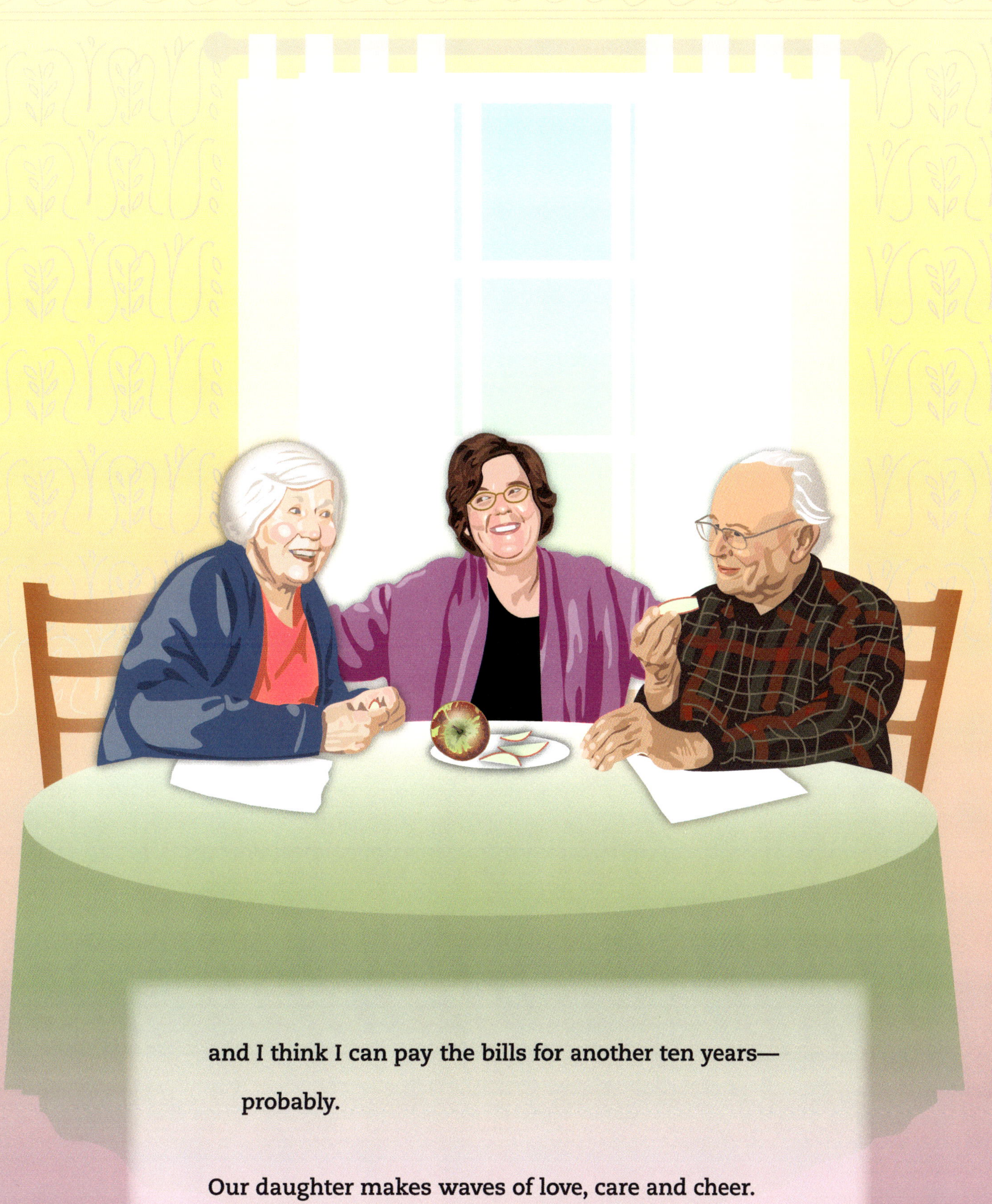

and I think I can pay the bills for another ten years—
     probably.

Our daughter makes waves of love, care and cheer.

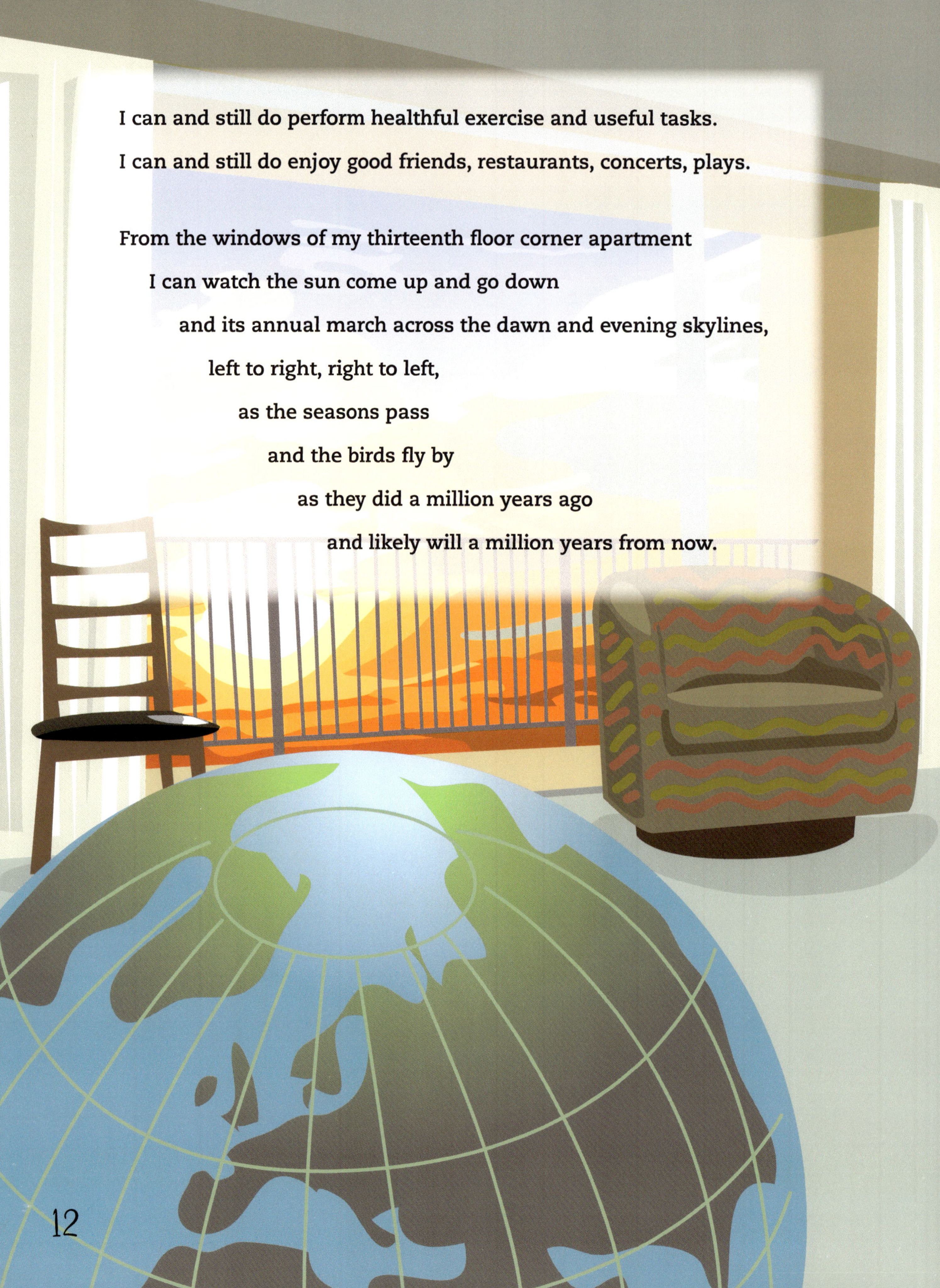

I can and still do perform healthful exercise and useful tasks.

I can and still do enjoy good friends, restaurants, concerts, plays.

From the windows of my thirteenth floor corner apartment

I can watch the sun come up and go down

and its annual march across the dawn and evening skylines,

left to right, right to left,

as the seasons pass

and the birds fly by

as they did a million years ago

and likely will a million years from now.

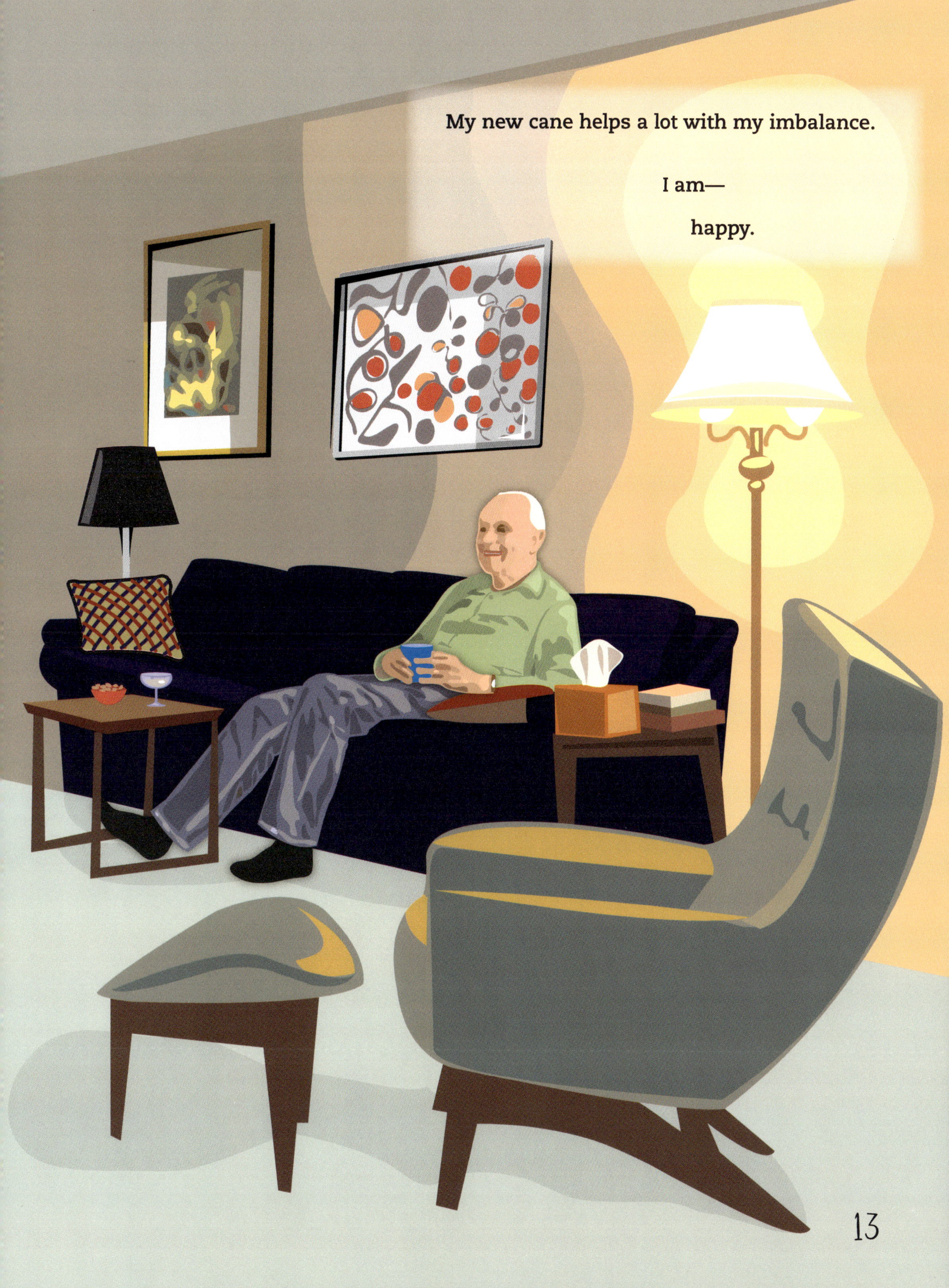

My new cane helps a lot with my imbalance.

I am—

happy.

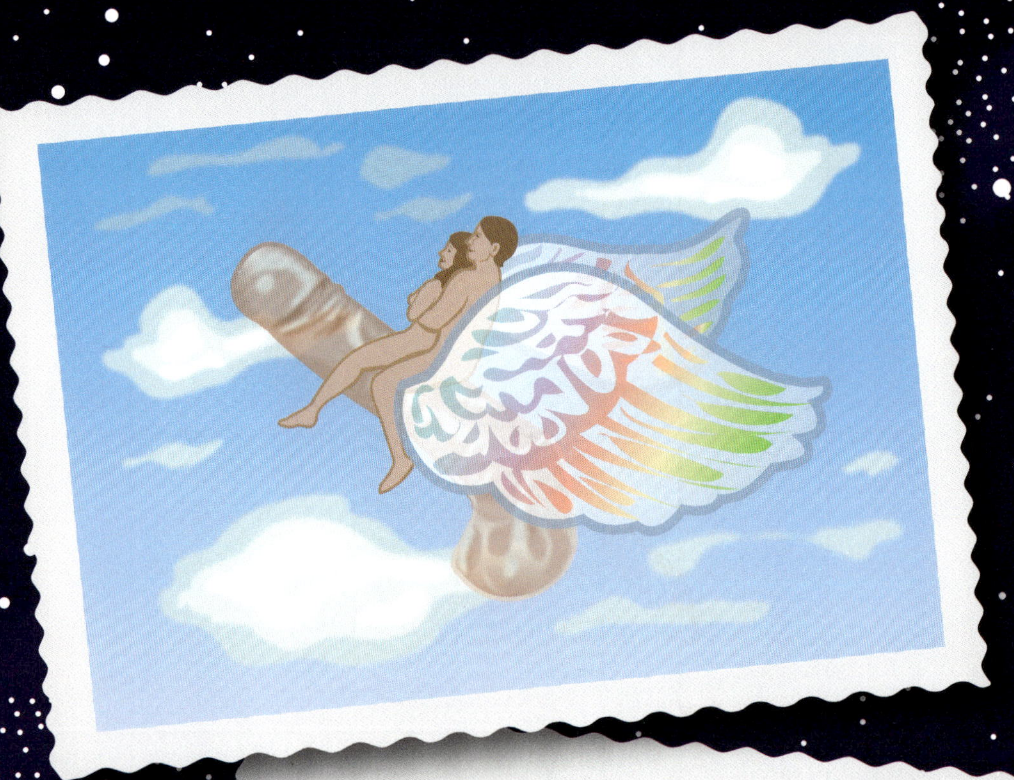

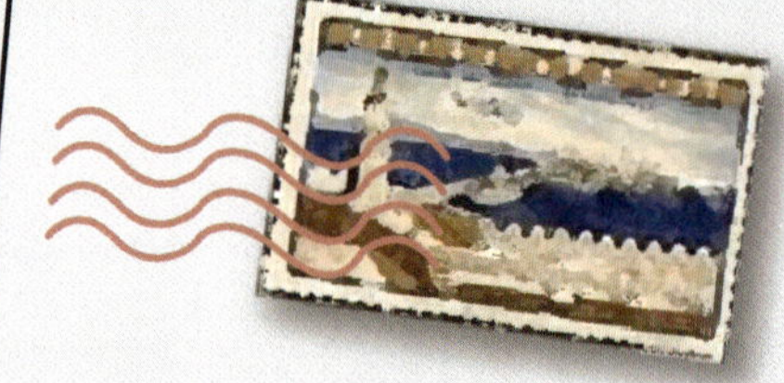

4/8/45

Hi Ray!
Today's history lesson —
the pleasures of the
ancient world! Bet you
never learned about this
in school — the classic
winged phallus of Pompeii
— first century A.D.
Will wonders never cease!

Cheers! Rob

Pfc. Raymond D. Watts,
33695383
Co. L, 303rd Inf. Regt.
A.P.O. 445
New York, N.Y.

The Dream

Hurry! I must write this down before it fades away.

It is 6:40 on Saturday morning.

My first pee wake-up last night was at 1 a.m.

My throat was a little sore when I went to sleep about 10.

Now it is a little sorer.

This is the familiar first sign of an oncoming cold.

I do the usual:

    swallow a whole gram of vitamin C with a whole glass of water.

I am soon back asleep.

Now it is 4:15 and my bladder again wakes me up.

The sore throat is a little better, but still there.

I take another 750 milligrams of the wonderful C vitamin

    and am soon again asleep.

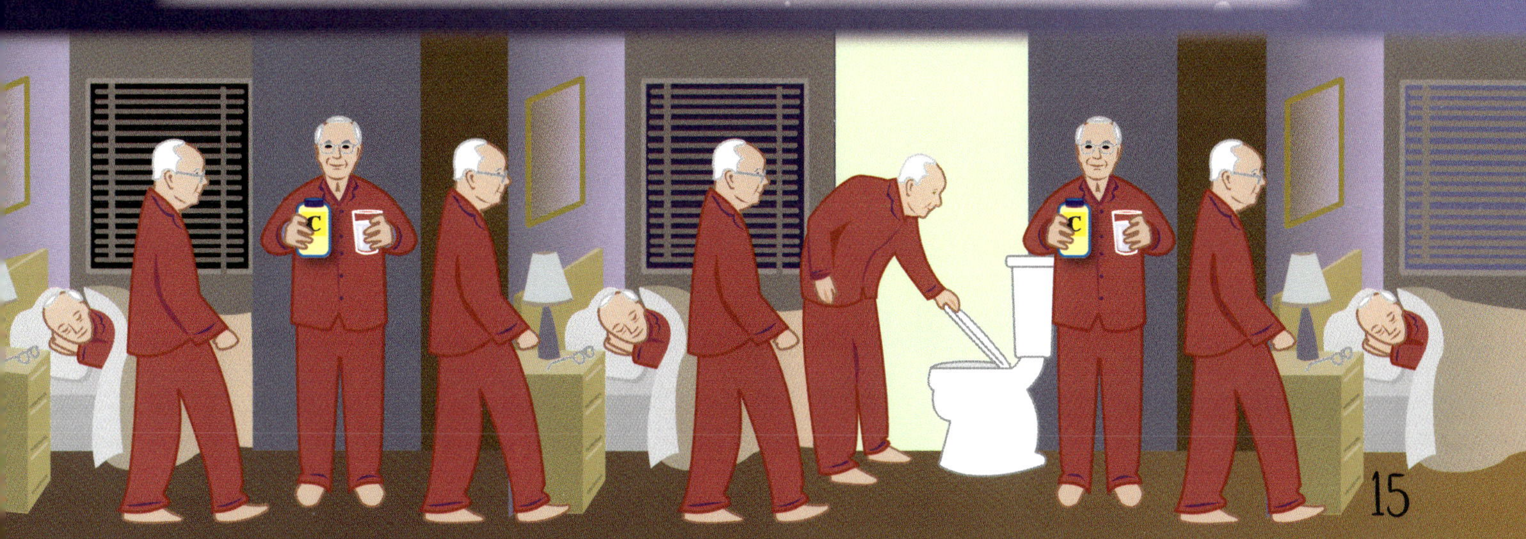

Then I am awake, it seems.

It's a summer day and I am walking with Penny,

    or maybe we're in a car.

Without words, outdoors in broad daylight with people passing by,

    we are hugging and kissing.

I feel my penis getting hard.

She reaches for it, briefly holds and pets it.

I say, "We need to get to bed."

She says nothing, but the answer is, "Yes."

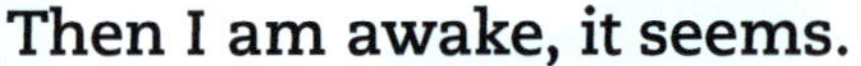

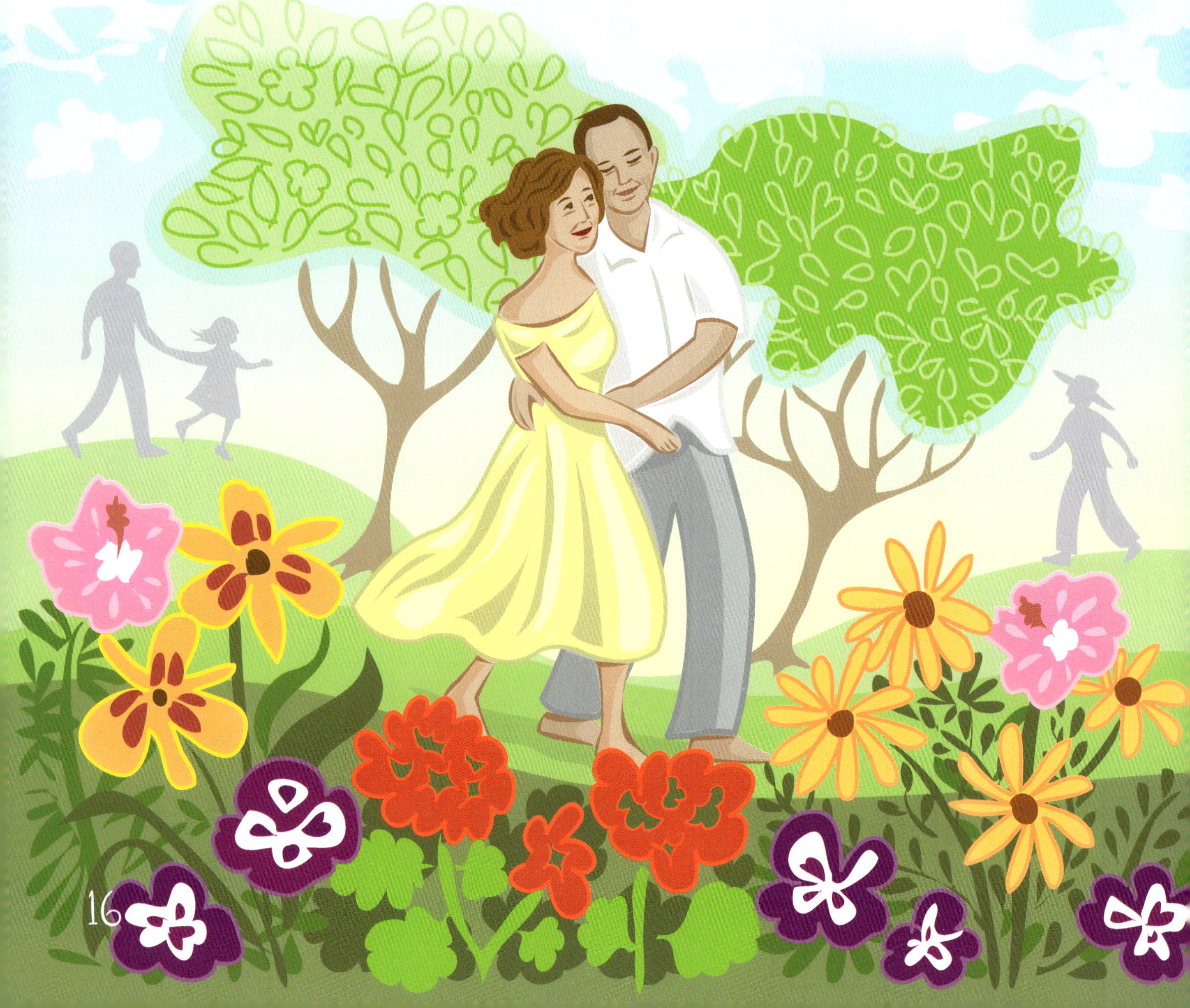

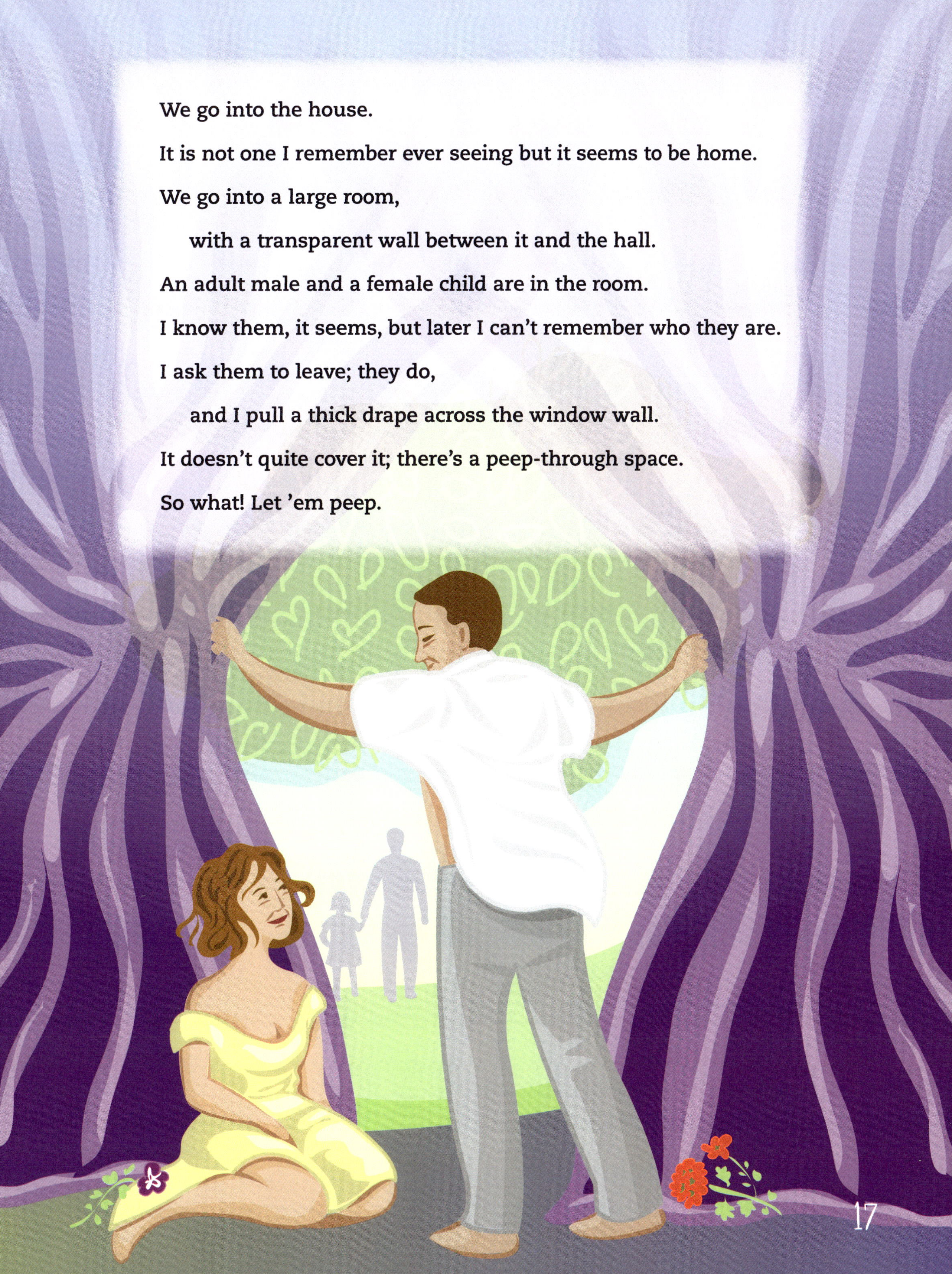

We go into the house.

It is not one I remember ever seeing but it seems to be home.

We go into a large room,

    with a transparent wall between it and the hall.

An adult male and a female child are in the room.

I know them, it seems, but later I can't remember who they are.

I ask them to leave; they do,

    and I pull a thick drape across the window wall.

It doesn't quite cover it; there's a peep-through space.

So what! Let 'em peep.

Penny and I quickly get into the large bed.

My penis has remained fully erect, hard.

Almost instantly it is inside her,

    although we are both still in our summer clothes.

Without ever disconnecting, I am able to open her shirt,

    caress and kiss her breasts.

Never uncoupling, we manage to become completely naked.

My phallus fills her vagina in a most delightful way.

The only thing wrong is that no orgasm comes;

    but it doesn't seem to matter to either of us.

We can wait.

We are so happy, so together, so in love.

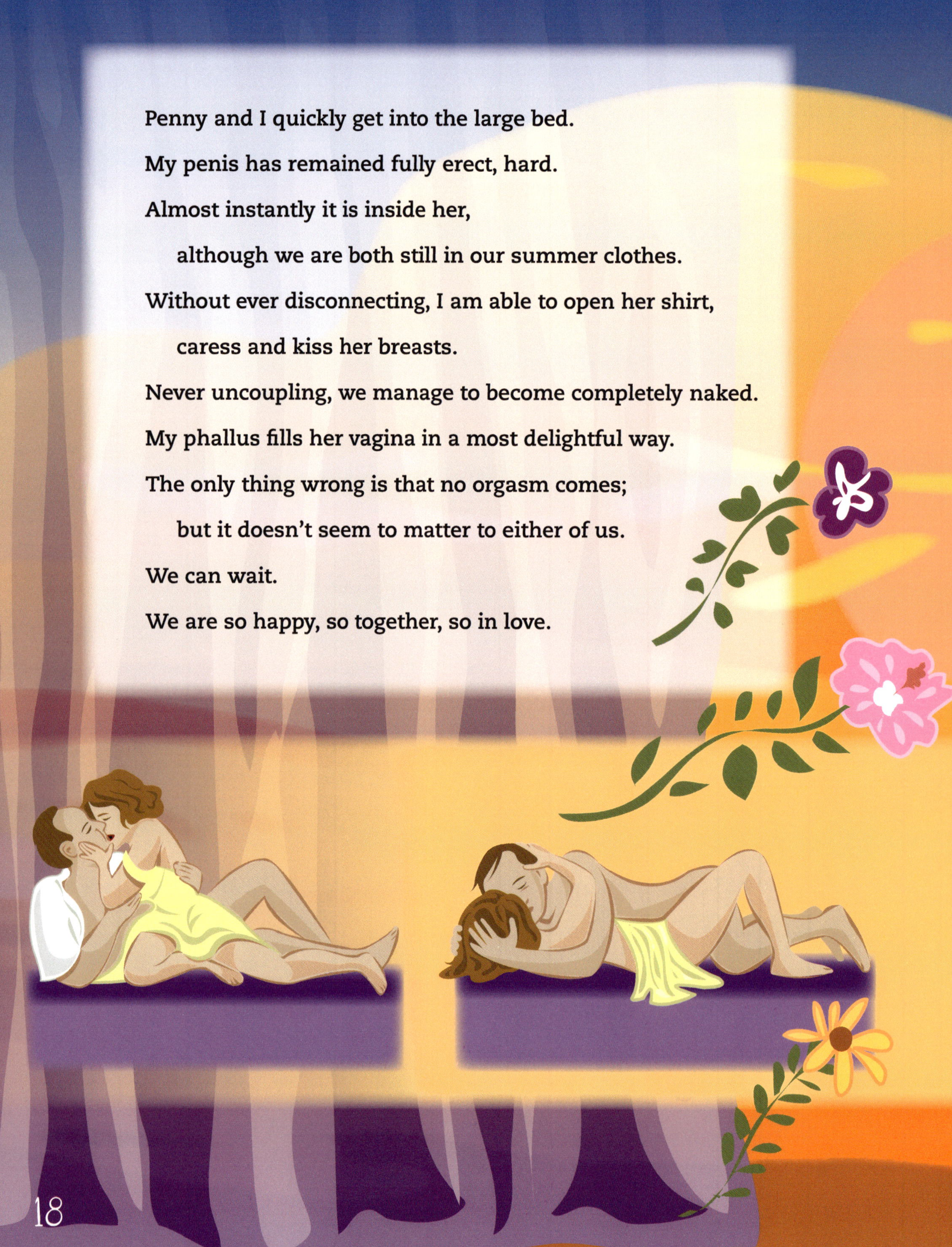

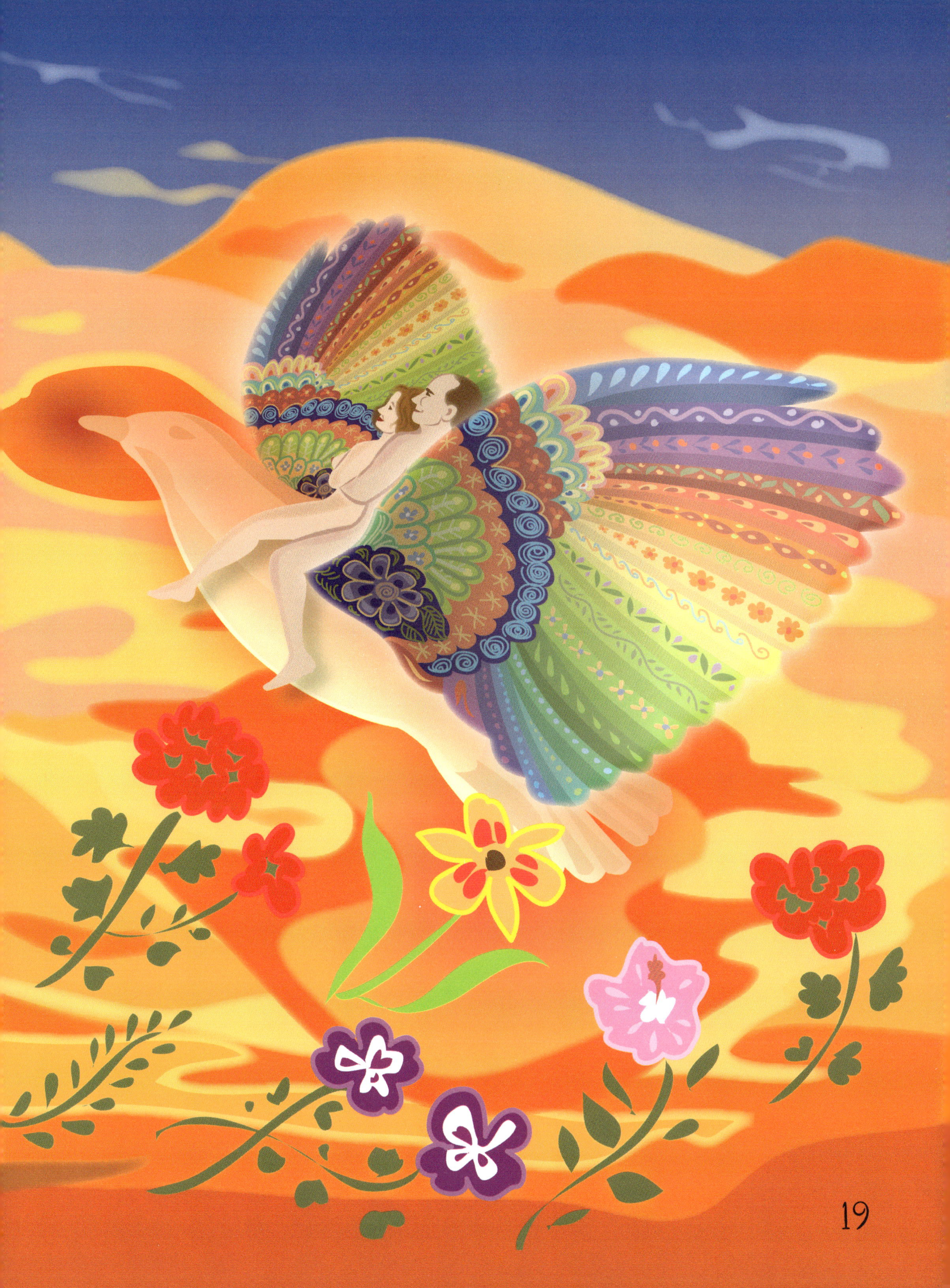

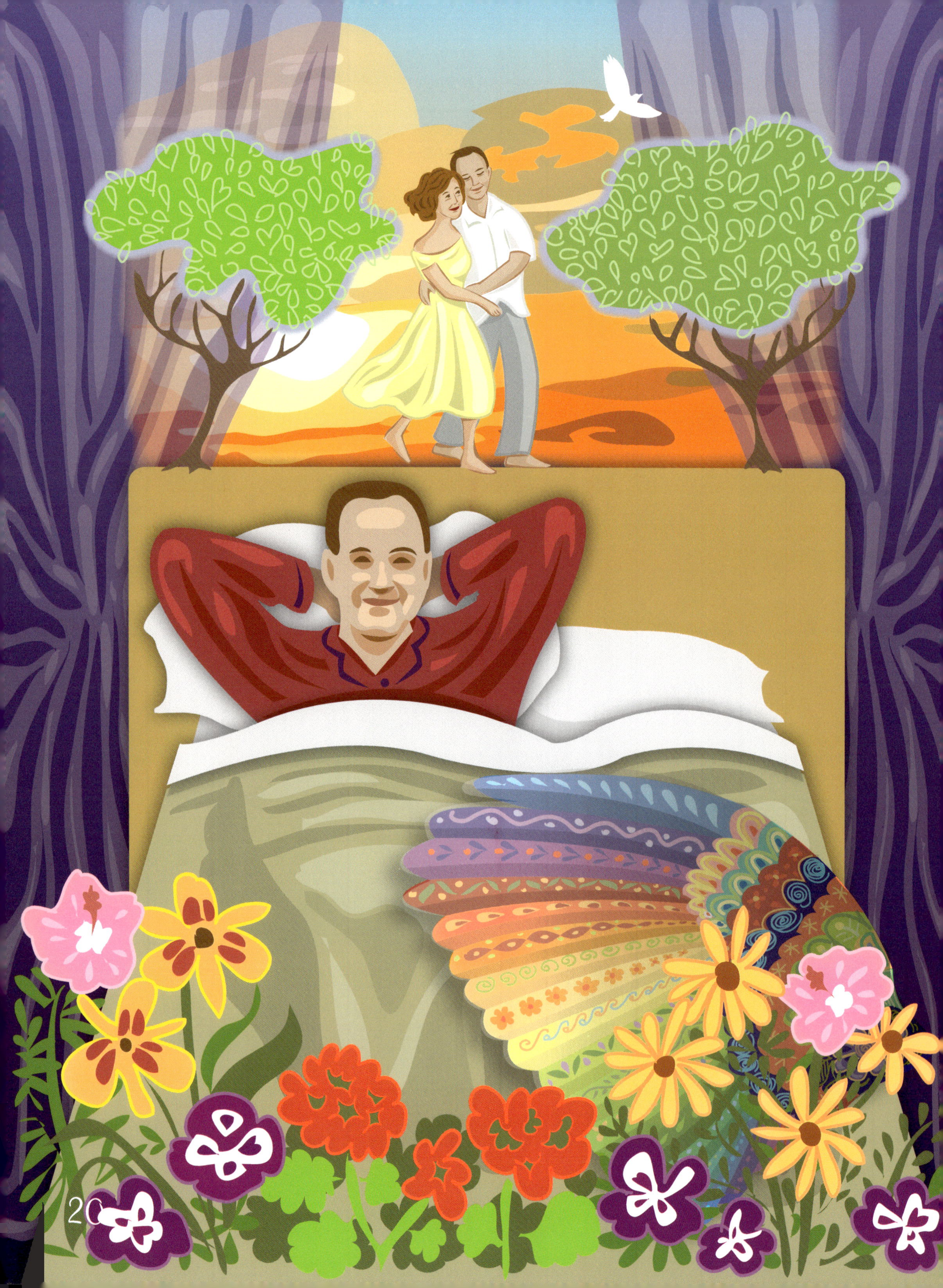

Then I *am* awake, alone in my dark bedroom in apartment 1310.

I am again small, flaccid and age 85,

    not the big, horny 50 of seconds ago;

        and Penny is once again gone, once again

            dead.

But I am just so damn happy!

What a beautiful gift is a good dream!

Waking from it I am

    for precious moments few but fervent

        remitted from frail 85 to fecund 50.

It is Nature's consolation prize for not giving me real magic,

    not giving me well-hung and life-lasting equipment

        for use in real extended youth with a living wife.

Now it is 7:20, and it is written.

I am so glad I got it down before I had time to forget.

The sore throat is better this morning;

    but cold or no cold, I'm hanging onto that vitamin C.

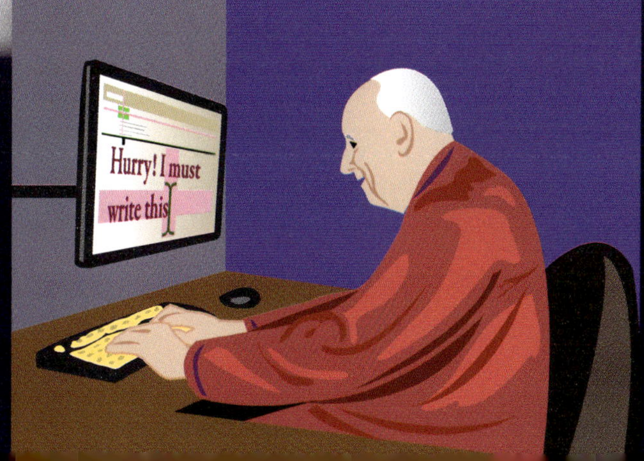

Sequel, Without Vitamin C

April 28, 2010

Now it is 6:30 a.m.

and I am again awaking from a remarkable dream.

I am outdoors in a treeless, barren landscape.

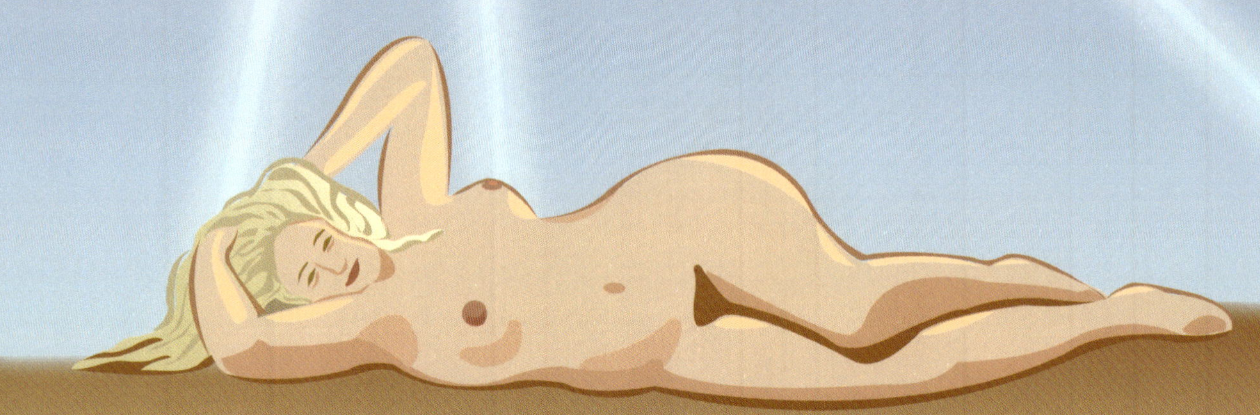

The sun is shining, the day warm but not hot.

The landscape is deserted—

   except for me and a woman

     I don't know and later can't clearly remember,

      except that she is white,

       neither pretty nor ugly,

        neither old nor young,

         neither fat nor skinny;

          but quite naked.

She is lying on the ground,

   which seems as soft and comfortable as a bed,

    awaiting me, with no apparent apprehension,

     pleasure or displeasure.

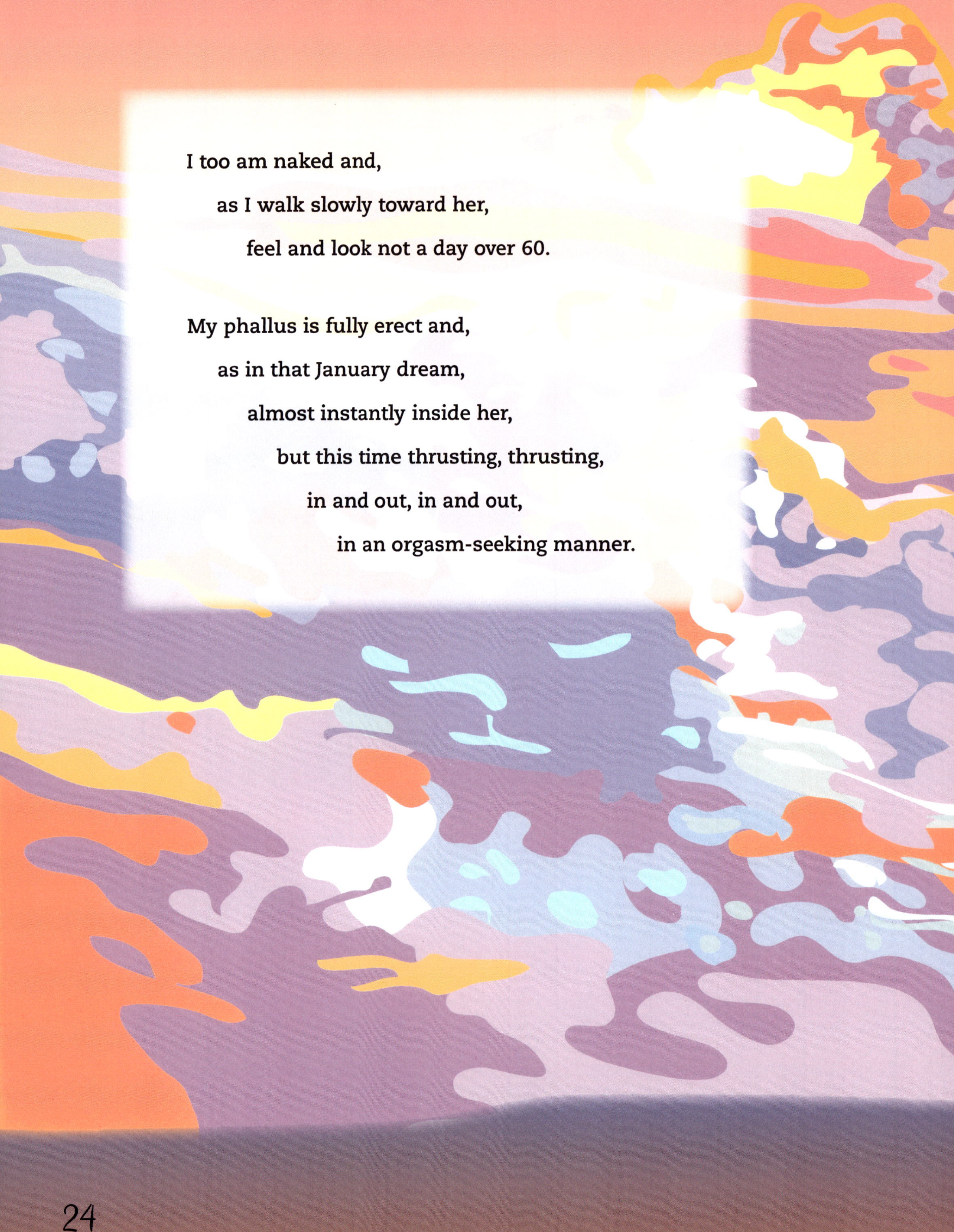

I too am naked and,

as I walk slowly toward her,

feel and look not a day over 60.

My phallus is fully erect and,

as in that January dream,

almost instantly inside her,

but this time thrusting, thrusting,

in and out, in and out,

in an orgasm-seeking manner.

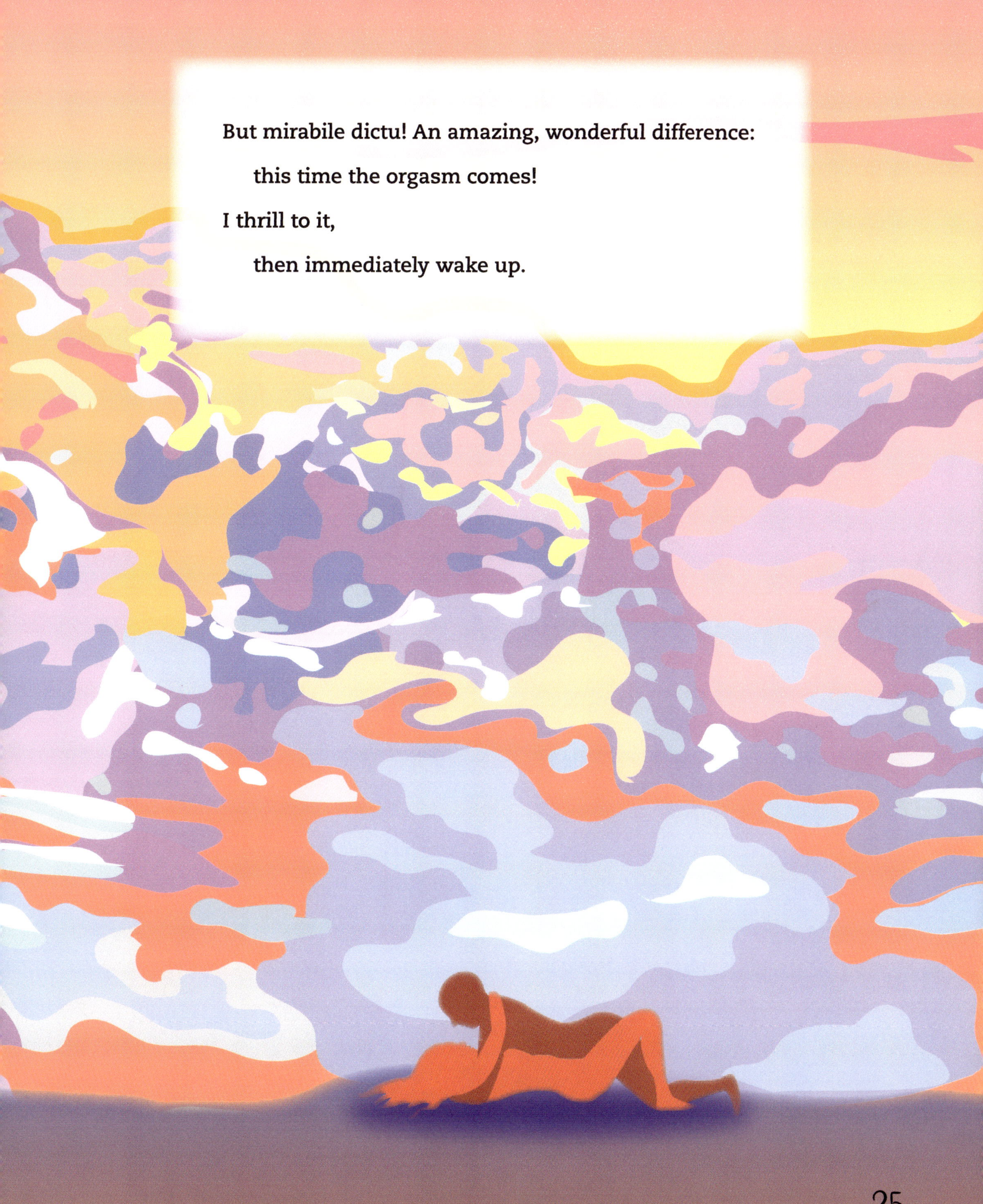
But mirabile dictu! An amazing, wonderful difference:
this time the orgasm comes!
I thrill to it,
then immediately wake up.

But, no wet dream, this; my diaper is dry,

    the orgasm, like the erection in this and the earlier dream,

        is entirely virtual—

            but realistic and oh so exciting.

No vitamin C, either.

Now I know, when I'm asleep and dreaming,

    both halves of that awful, sad line in *OLD AGE*

        have become untrue.

Let's hear it for the brain's wonderful memory cells!

From here on out in what remains of my long life

    I shall (virtually) meditate, pray and chant

        for repetitions of such dreams,

            as early and often

                as God, Jesus, Karma, Nature (or whatever)

                will vouchsafe me.

But next time, please,

    could The Force, The Dream Giver,

        again make the woman be Penny?

Amen.

My Prayer Is Answered

After a day of satisfying work alone, I go to bed early, about 9:30.

As an ophthalmologist has recommended,

   I have first washed my eyelids with baby soap,

      then lain down with a hot compress over my eyes.

It must have rung long and loud,

   but I never heard the five-minute timer.

Instead, with no sense of time, travel, distance or magic,

   I am in another bed, another room, another house—

      and much younger.

And *Penny* is with me!

Our two bodies are entwined, combined,

   and, between them both,

      encumbered with only one garment.

It is her bra.

That is desirable, even necessary.

My deliberate, fumbling unhooking and removal

   of that romantic device

      is an important part of our accustomed foreplay.

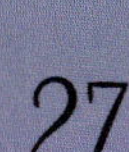

The foreplay goes on a long time.

It is very thorough, very exciting.

My phallus all the while is proudly, firmly erect.

The dear hand of my darling guides it to penetration.

Our coupling also lasts and lasts,

    but (nothing is perfect!) no orgasm comes,

        at least not to me.

I am still striving, energetically, to remedy that

    when the vision ends.

I am awake just long enough for the dream briefly to register,

    then fall back asleep

        for so long that delicious details grow fuzzy.

At 11:30 I am fully awake, needing to pee,

    displeased to find a cold damp washcloth over my face,

        but only a bit surprised to be again 86 years old,

          flaccid and alone.

But wotthehell!

My prayer has been answered!

Penny returned to my dream, my bed!

I am happy; once again, I am happy.

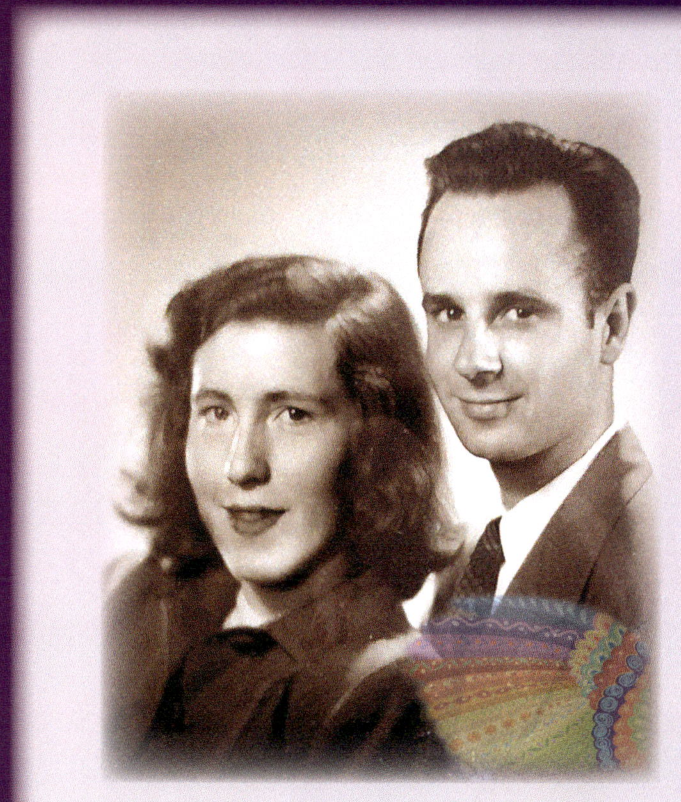

Penny and Ray in 1948

Photo by Axel Bahnsen

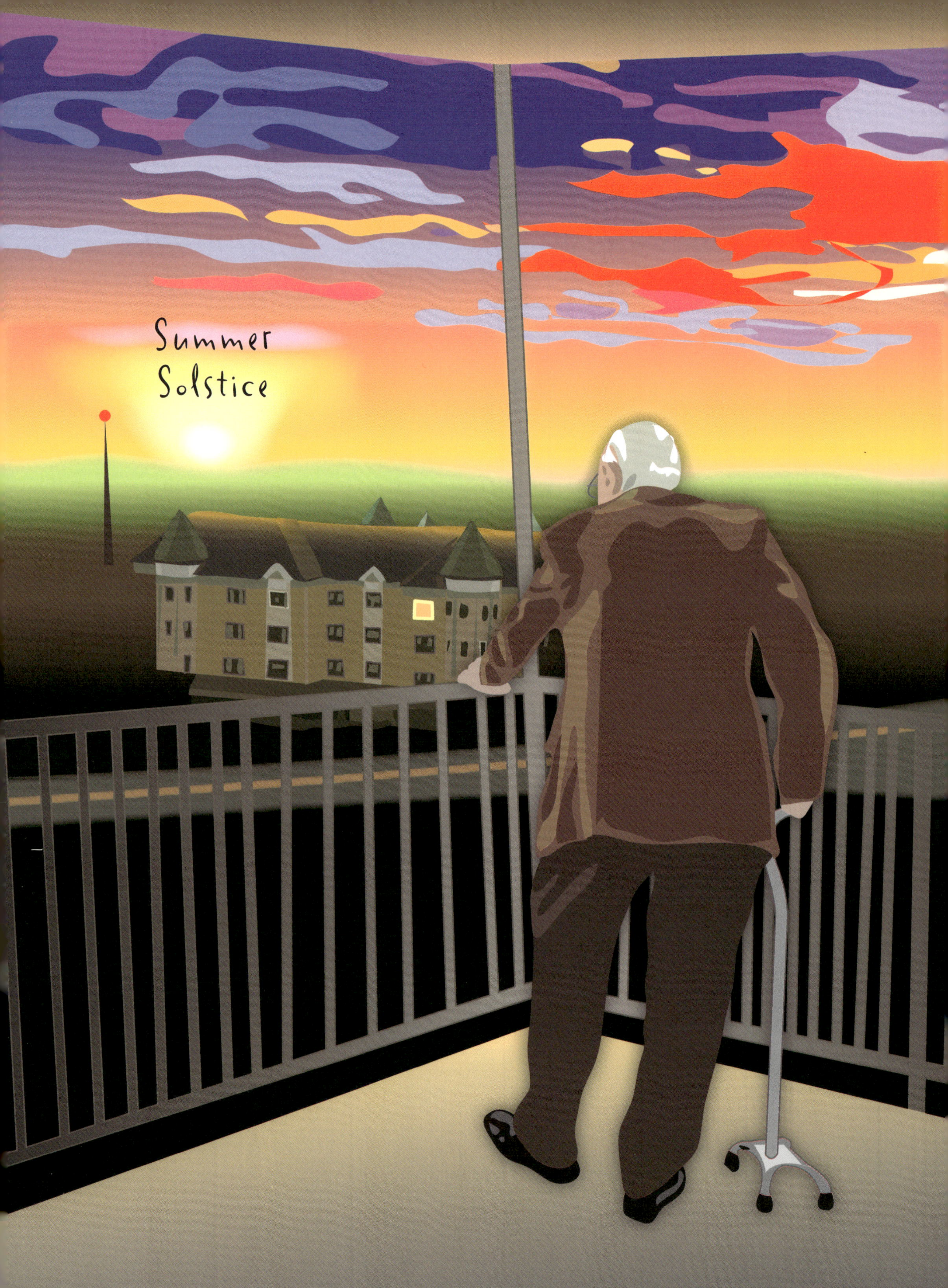
Summer
Solstice

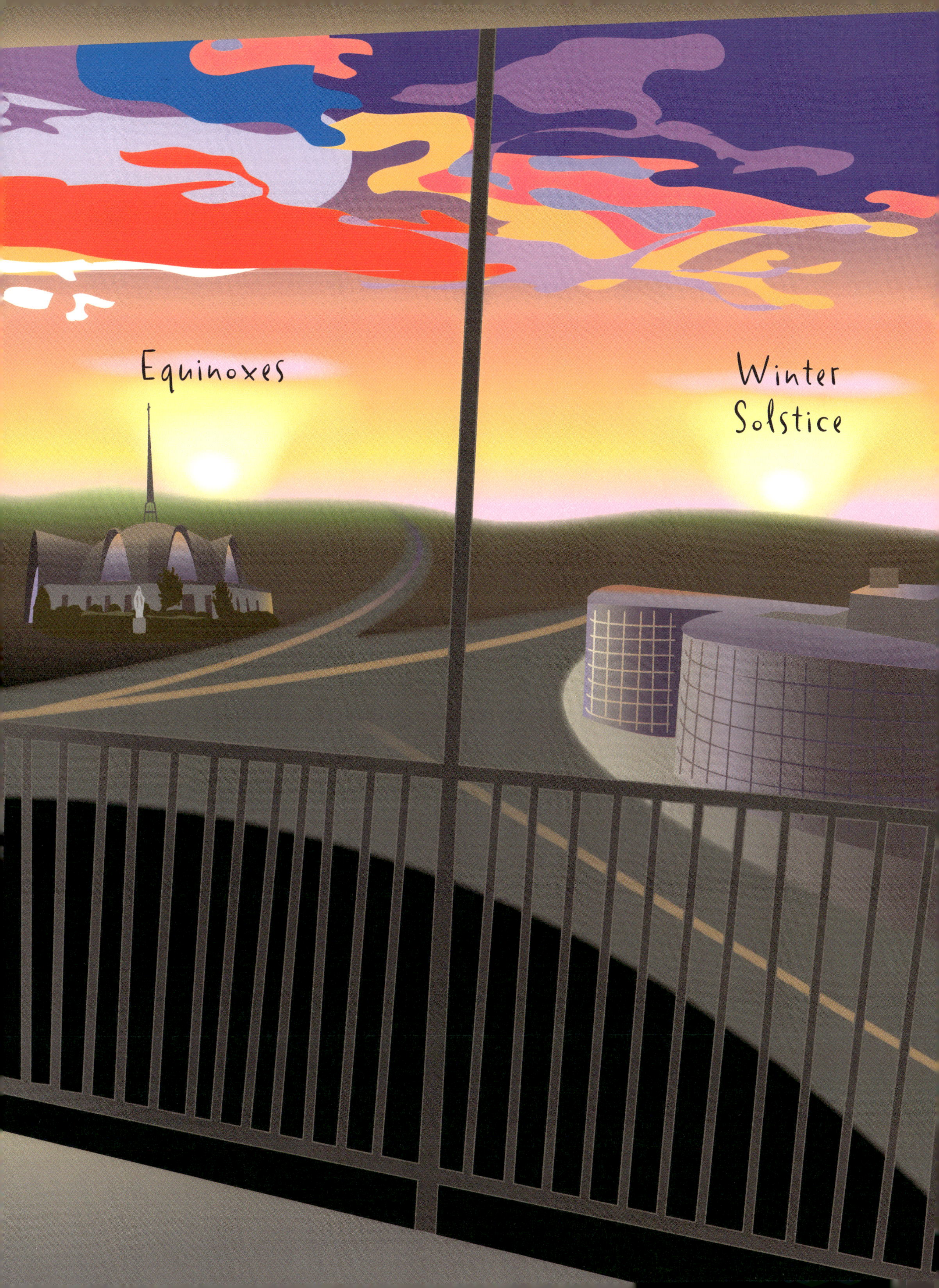

Equinoxes
Winter
Solstice

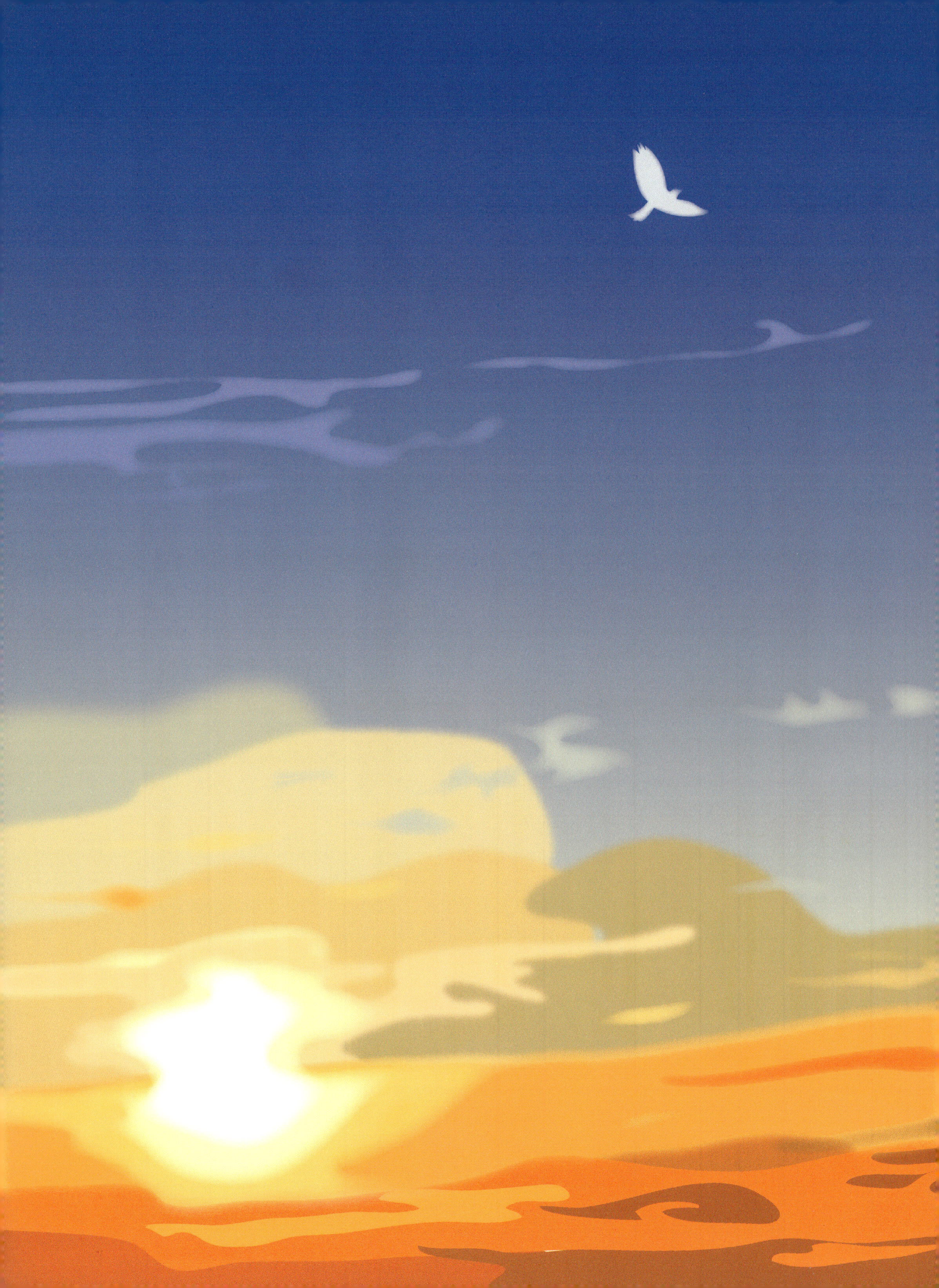

CPSIA information can be obtained
at www.ICGtesting.com
Printed in the USA
246079LV00006B